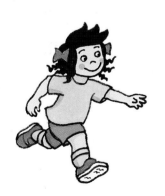

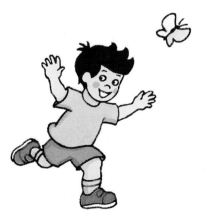

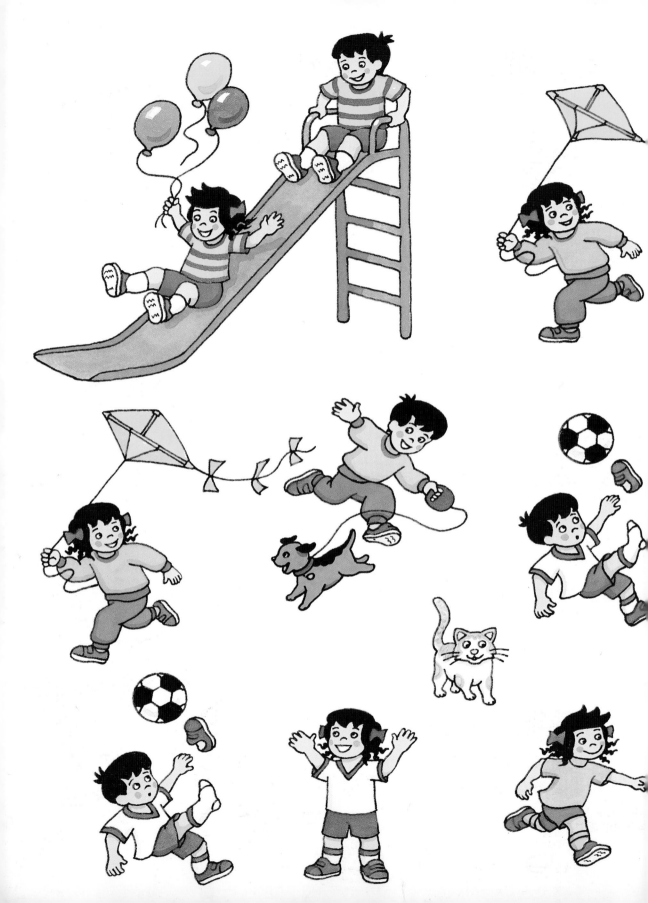

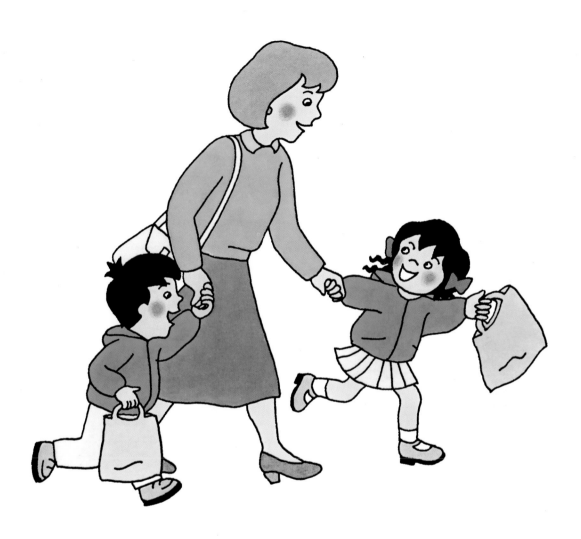

One morning Topsy and Tim were
in a great hurry to get to school.
'The police are coming to talk
to us today,' they told Mummy.

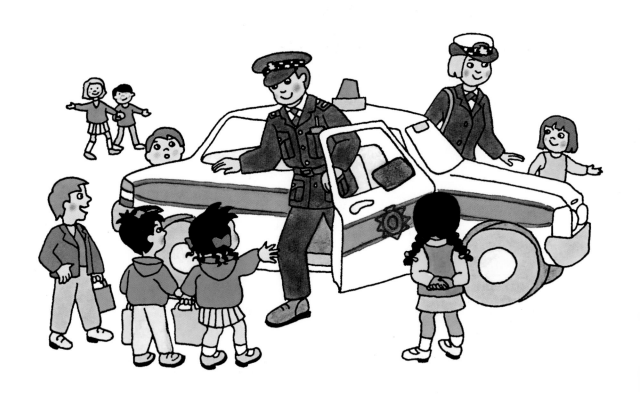

When they reached school a
police car was already there.
A policeman and a policewoman
got out.
'Can anyone tell us where to find
Miss Terry?' they asked.
'Why? What's she done?' said
Andy Anderson.

Topsy and Tim knew where
to find Miss Terry.
'Miss Terry is our teacher,'
they said.

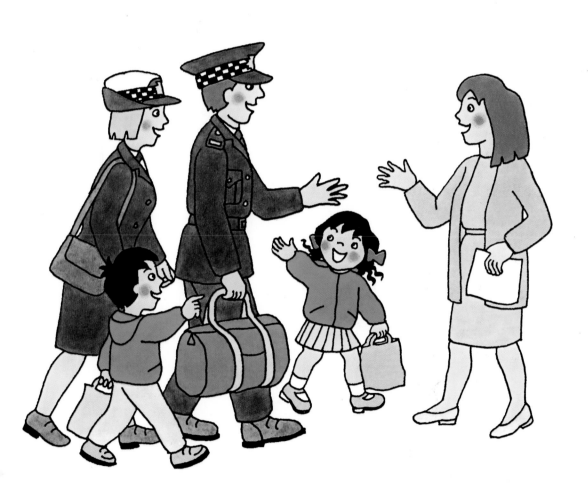

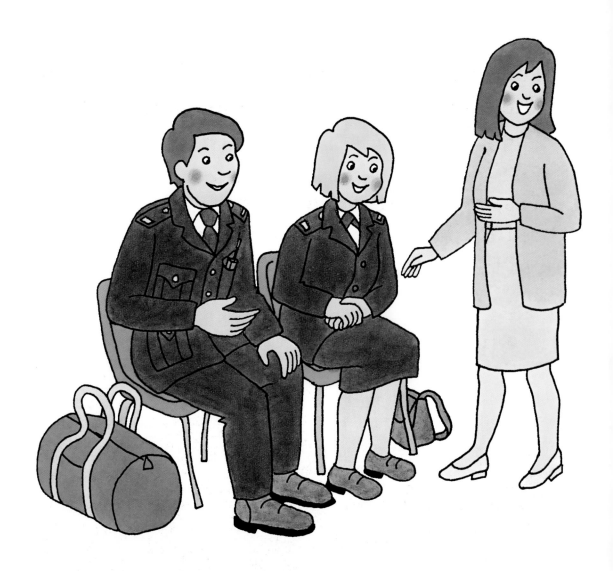

'Police Constable Webb and Woman
Police Constable May have come
to tell us all about the work
that the police do,' said Miss Terry.
'Do any of you children know the
jobs that the police do?'

'They catch burglars,' said Andy Anderson.
'They look after traffic,' said Tim.
'They find you when you are lost,'
said Topsy.
'Yes, we do all those things,'
said PC Webb, 'and we look after
lost things as well as lost children.'

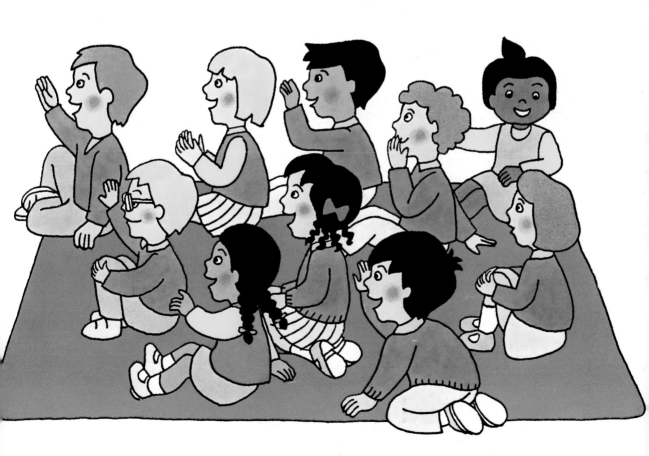

'Suppose Tim was walking down
the street,' said PC Webb, 'and
he found a purse full of money
on the ground. What should he do?'
'Spend it?' said Andy Anderson.
'No,' said PC Webb. 'That would
be very wrong. He should take it
to a police station.'

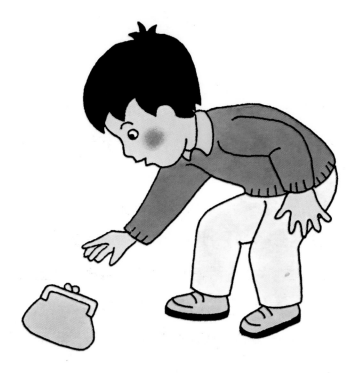

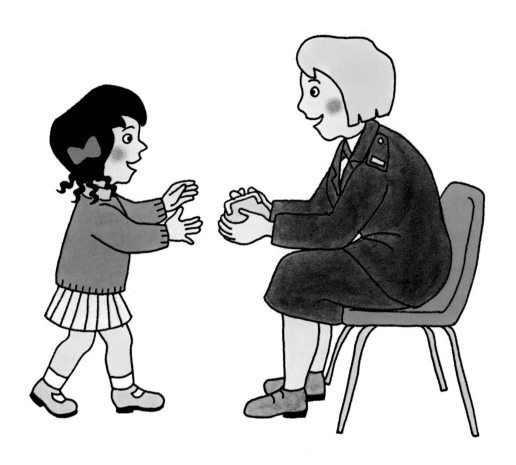

'Suppose Topsy was the one who
had lost the purse,' said WPC May.
'What should she do?'
None of the children knew.
'She should go to the police station
and tell them she had lost her purse,'
said WPC May. 'Then the police
would be able to give it back to her.'

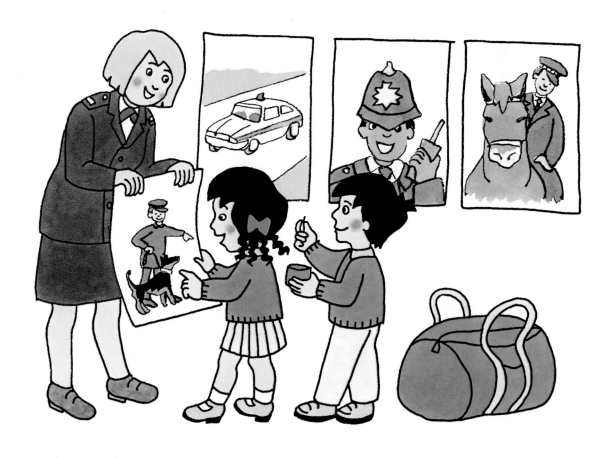

WPC May asked Topsy and Tim
to help her pin up some pictures
of the police at work.
One of the pictures showed a police dog.
'Have you got a police dog?' asked Topsy.

'No,' said WPC May. 'Police dogs belong to police dog handlers. The dogs are trained to find things that are lost or hidden. They are very clever.'

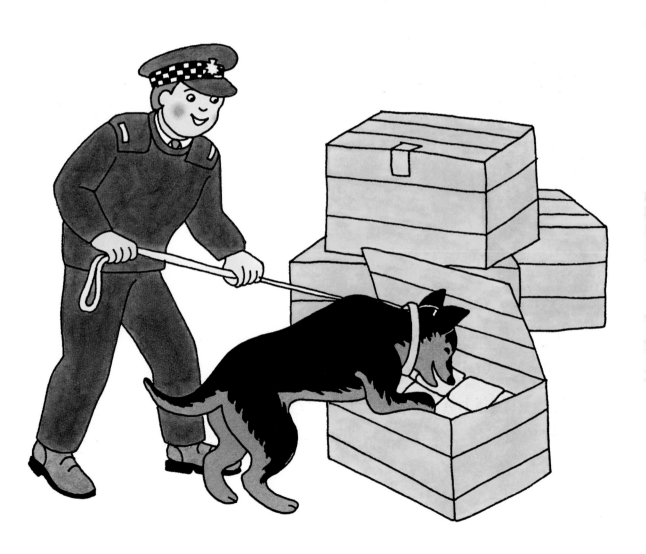

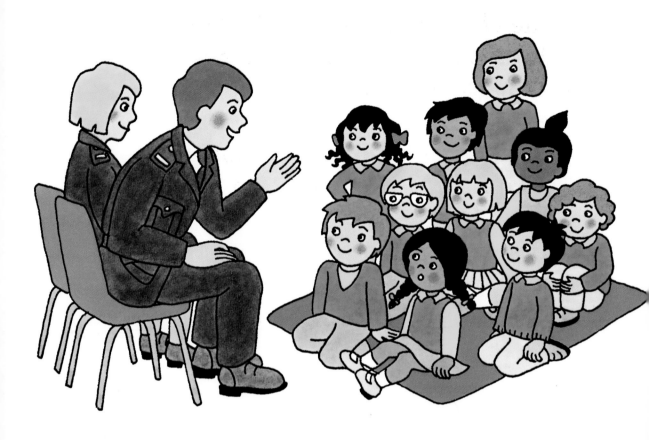

PC Webb told the children that
one of the most important jobs
the police do is to come into
schools and talk to children
about safety.
'Some places are dangerous to play in,'
he said.

The children helped PC Webb
think of some dangerous places.
'Don't play near deep water —
you might fall in,' said Kerry.
'Don't play by a railway line —
a train might hit you,' said
little Stevie Dunton.
'Don't play on a building site —
you could cut yourself on something
sharp and rusty,' said Louise Lewis.

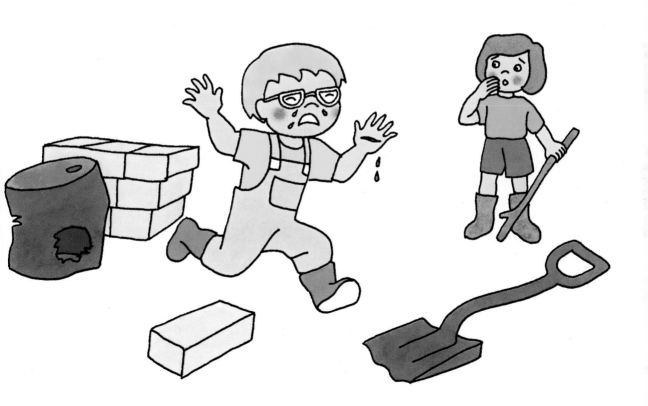

'Always stay where your mother can keep an eye on you,' said PC Webb, 'and never ever talk to strangers. If a stranger tries to talk to you in the street or anywhere else, don't let them come near you.'
'What is a stranger?' asked Tim.

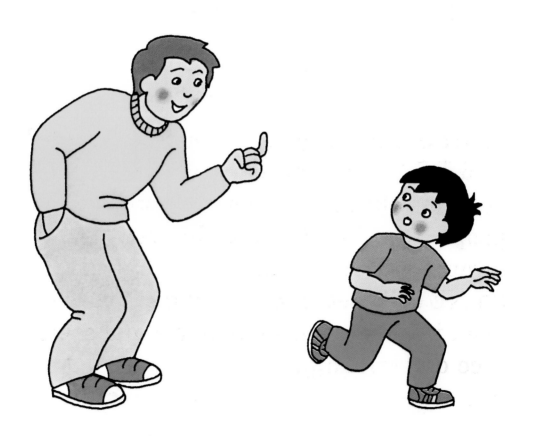

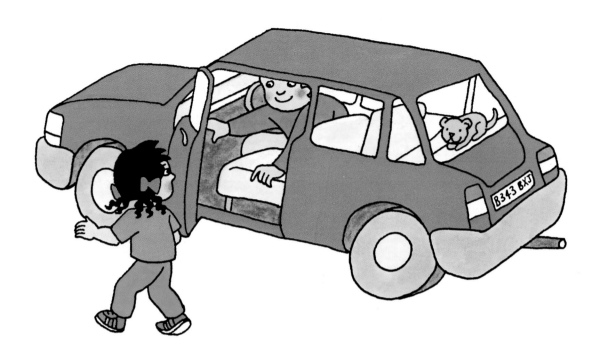

'A stranger is someone you don't know,'
said PC Webb. 'Most people are
good and kind, but there are some
people who like to take children
away and hurt them.
So NEVER get into a stranger's car —
even if they know your name and seem
nice and friendly.'

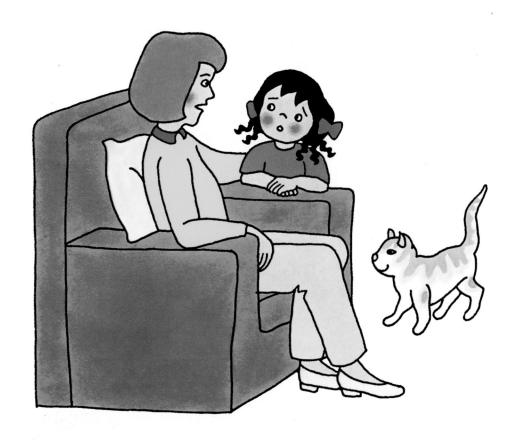

'If a stranger has tried to talk
to you, or asked you to get in
his car, tell your mummy or your
teacher and they should tell the
police,' said PC Webb.

WPC May helped the children
act a play called Stranger-Danger.
Andy Anderson was a bad stranger.
'Will you help me find my
lost puppy?' he said to Vinda.
'No!' shouted Vinda, keeping
out of his way.

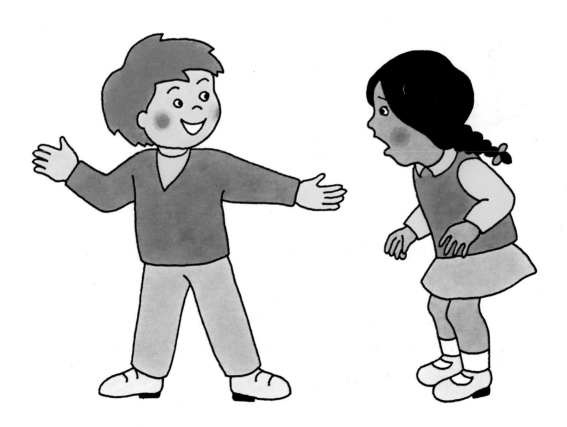

Rai was Vinda's daddy.
He took Vinda to the police station
to see WPC Topsy and PC Tim.
'My little girl says a stranger
frightened her,' said Rai.
'Thank you for telling us,' said Tim.
'We will try and catch that bad man.'

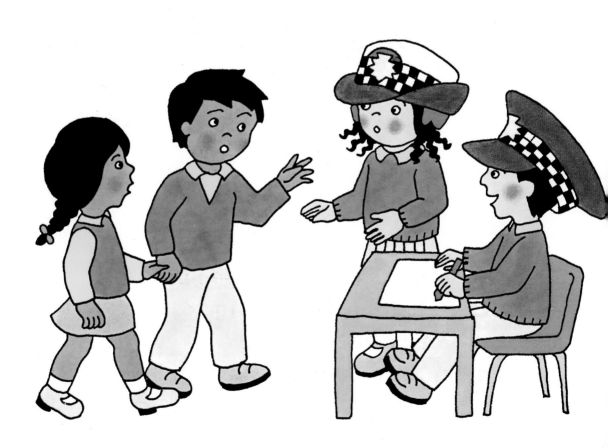

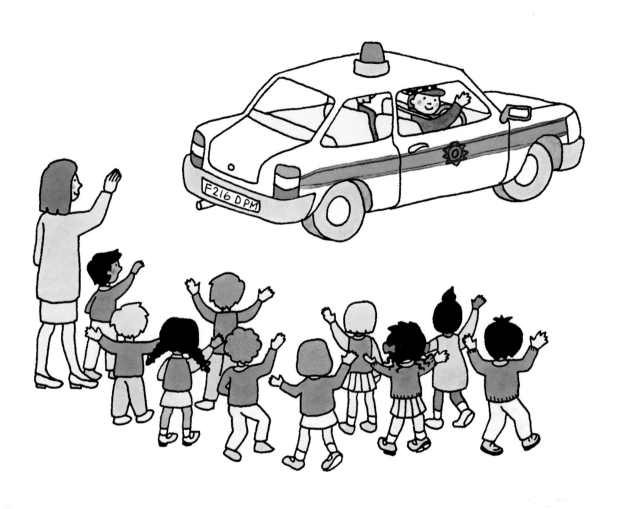

After the play it was time for
PC Webb and WPC May to go back
to their police station.
The children waved goodbye.

On their way home from school
that day Topsy saw something shiny
on the pavement. It was a very
pretty brooch.
'Someone will be sad to have lost
such a nice brooch,' said Mummy.

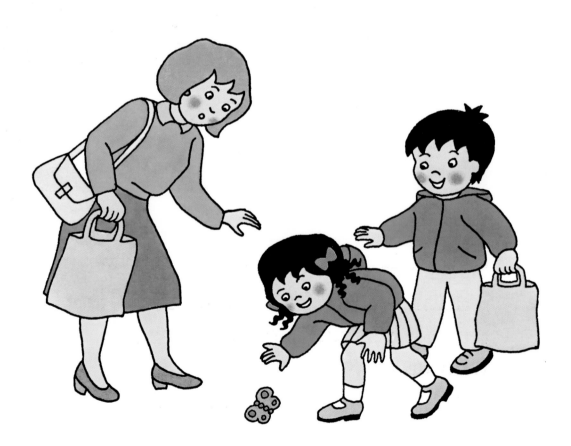

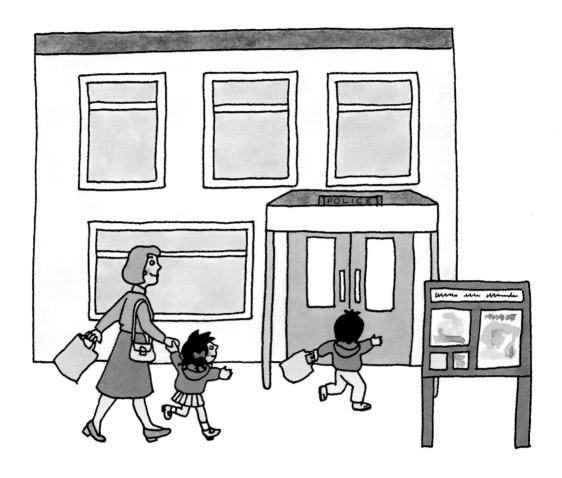

'We must take it to the police
station,' said Tim. 'Then the police
can give it back to the person
who lost it.'

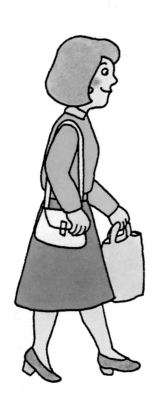
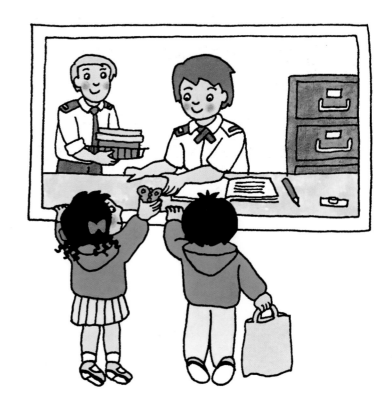

'Hello,' said the desk sergeant in
the police station. 'Can I help you?'
'Topsy's found a pretty brooch,'
said Tim. The desk sergeant took
the brooch and wrote about it
in her book. She wrote down Topsy
and Tim's address too.
'We will let you know if we find
the owner,' she said.

They went home and were having tea
when the phone rang. Dad answered it.
It was the police to say that they
had found the owner of the lost brooch.
'I wonder who it belonged to?' said
Mummy.

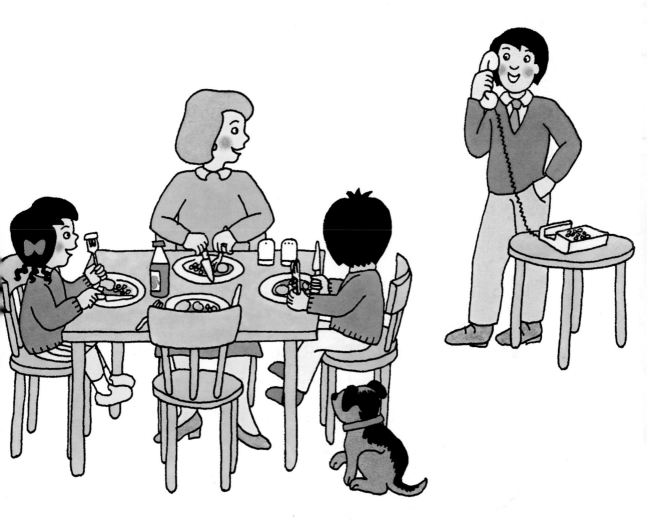

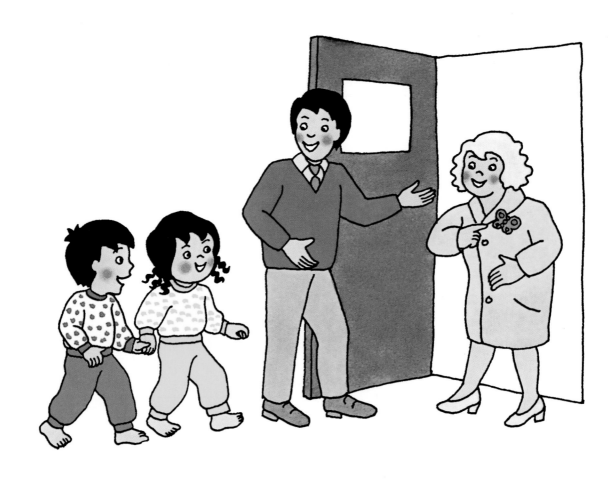

That night, when Topsy and Tim
were getting ready for bed, there
was a knock at the door. It was
Mrs Higley-Pigley.
'Thank you, Topsy and Tim,' she said,
'for finding my very special brooch
and for taking it to the police.'

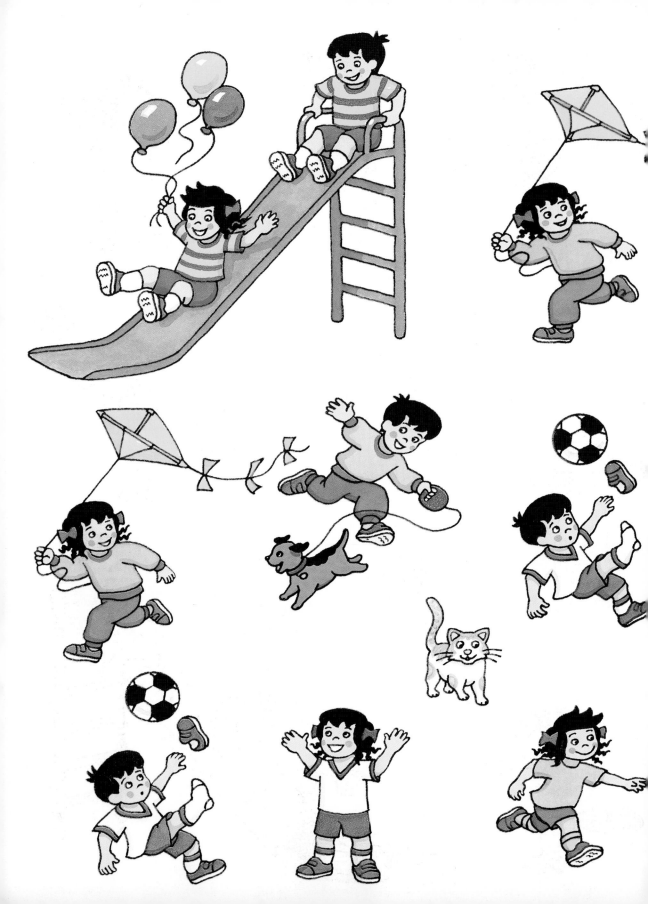

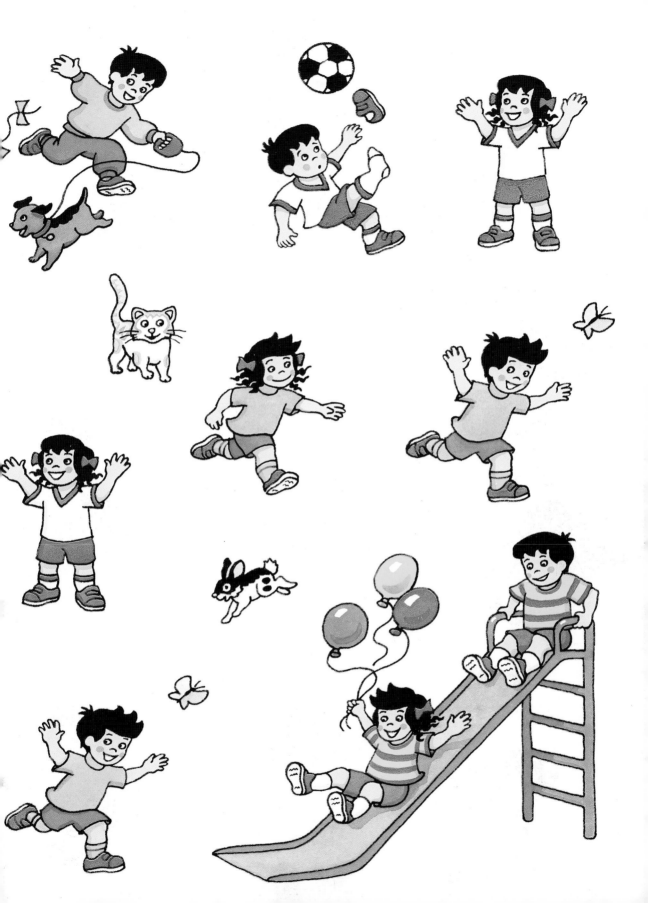